Bodyweight Training For Cycling

By Matt Schifferle

Text Copyright © 2018 Matthew J. Schifferle
All Rights Reserved

ISBN-13: 978-1727603149

ISBN-10: 1727603141

The information provided in this book is designed to provide helpful information on the subjects discussed. This book is not meant to be used, nor should it be used, to diagnose or treat any medical condition. For diagnosis or treatment of any medical problem, consult your own physician. The publisher and author are not responsible for any specific health or allergy needs that may require medical supervision and are not liable for any damages or negative consequences from any treatment, action, application or preparation, to any person reading or following the information in this book. References are provided for informational purposes only and do not constitute endorsement of any websites or other sources. Readers should be aware that the websites listed in this book may change.

Cover photo and design by Chris Clemens at
http://www.thinkpilgrim.com

Dedicated to my best friend and teammate, Chris Niggel. Thank you for helping me keep the rubber side down at least in life if not always on the bike.

Table of Contents

INTRODUCTION	5
CHAPTER 1 WHY USE STRENGTH TRAINING?	6
CHAPTER 2 THREE MOVES FOR ULTIMATE PERFORMANCE	14
CHAPTER 3 TWO MOVES FOR TOTAL CONTROL	36
CHAPTER 4 ACCESSORY MOVES	41
CHAPTER 5 SIMPLE STRETCHES FOR AN EASIER RIDE	45
CHAPTER 6 ROUTINES AND TRAINING TIPS FOR SUCCESS	50

Introduction

This book was written for the single purpose to help you ride your bike, longer, faster and better while having more fun with every pedal stroke. Whether you're a criterium warrior, a single track bomber, or a die-hard commuter the exercises in this book will help you ride at your very best for years to come.

Unlike other exercise programs, this exercise approach isn't supposed to be a focal point of your fitness plan or a lifestyle. It's a supplemental form of training that will enhance your most essential training which is riding your bike. Like the bicycle itself, everything within these pages is designed for efficiency and is free of nonessential fluff that can weigh down your training program.

Okay, that's enough of an introduction let's get right down to business with understanding why this sort of training significantly improves your ability to ride, what exercises you'll be practicing and a few basic routines that will deliver the results you want.

The best ride of your life is still out there, and this book will help you find it. Let's suit up, clip in and get started.

-Matt Schifferle

Chapter 1

Why Use Strength Training?

These days, strength training is seen as a necessary part of an athlete's training program. Even grade-school athletes are involved in rigorous workout programs, and it seems like there's a strength and conditioning gym on every street corner. It may seem obvious now, but the idea of practicing strength exercises to improve athletic performance, or even endurance, is a somewhat new idea.

Back in the 1960's a scrappy young guy named Bruce Lee started to supplement his martial arts training with weight lifting techniques that he learned from local bodybuilders. At the time, lifting weights to improve physical performance was a pretty revolutionary idea. Critics claimed lifting would make athletes "muscle bound" and slow. Building big muscles was supposedly all show and no go.

Those critics weren't entirely wrong. Strength training is much like medicine. It certainly can wreak havoc on your athletic performance if you don't know how to use it correctly. However, if you apply it in the right dose, it can provide massive benefits such as:

#1 It adds horsepower to your engine

As a cyclist, your muscles are your engine. Even the most high-tech racing bikes are only as fast as the person that's turning the pedals. This is why adding even a little extra strength can improve everything from your ability to climb up steep mountain passes to technical control over rough terrain.

#2 It helps correct imbalances and chronic problems

Highly repetitive activities can increase the risk of chronic problems like muscle imbalances and stiffness. Cycling is one of the riskiest forms of exercise since it involves sitting hunched over which is already something many people do too much in daily life.

These muscle imbalances can cause all sorts of problems from weaknesses, poor posture, chronic pain and even poor performance. Unfortunately, refraining from such detrimental habits does little to correct these issues. Once your body creates a habitual imbalance, it's there to stay even if you never sit in a chair or ride a bike ever again. the good news is you can reverse pesky imbalances through using corrective strength exercises. You can even restore muscle balance if you continue to sit at a desk all day and ride all weekend.

#3 It complements the benefits of cycling

Cycling is a fantastic form of exercise, but It's not perfect. Like all exercises, it has its weaknesses and shortcomings. Strength training fills in the conditioning gaps that pedal pushing fails to address. Shoring up these weaknesses helps you ride at your best while adding longevity to your cycling career.

So the whole idea of using strength training to enhance your cycling is a pretty good idea since it can potentially bring you many benefits, however there is a potential downside. Strength training, especially with heavy weights, can be costly and tedious. It can also put you at risk of injury if you don't know what you're doing. That's why bodyweight strength training can be such a perfect fit for cycling.

Why Use Calisthenics?

Strength training is excellent, but I don't blame anyone for turning away from weightlifting especially when their focus is on endurance disciplines like cycling. Biking requires a lot of time, energy and often money, so it's hard to justify spending even more resources to build muscle and strength. Heavy lifting can also handicap your performance. I found this out the hard way when I started lifting weights after a successful racing career in college.

My story

As a kid, I'd always loved riding my bike around my neighborhood as fast as possible. In college, I joined the U.V.M Cycling Club where I raced mountain bikes in the fall and road bikes in the spring. I spent the summer training in local Wednesday 20K mountain bike races.

By my senior year, I had worked up from a back-of-the-pack C-class racer to a consistent top-ten B-class contender with some podiums and even a few wins under my belt. I was also completing the 20K training races in under an hour. I was at the peak of my racing career and felt great, but there were some slow and frustrating years just ahead.

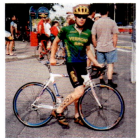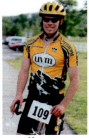

At 150 pounds I was at the peak of my collegiate racing career.

After graduating, I still rode my bike 2-3 times a week and I continued to race in the weekly training races over the summer. Despite my continued love for cycling I had to admit that I was no longer a bike racer. I was just a guy who raced his bike. That was okay though because I was quickly falling in love with my new obsession; strength training.

I had heard the cautionary tales of what would happen to my performance if I gained too much muscle weight. Fellow cyclists told me I would become slow and heavy if I packed on too much muscle. I figured I might get a little slower, but how bad could it be? It turned out my friends were 100% correct.

My 25-year-old muscles responded quickly to lifting, and I packed on 20 pounds in just 6 months. Almost all of it was from my waist up as I made the mistake of believing that riding alone was enough to make my legs as strong enough. The extra weight, coupled with less time on the bike, hit my training race times hard. By the end of the following season, my lap times had swollen by well over 70 minutes.

Eventually, I wised up and started doing strength work for my legs which helped, but not much. My race performance continued to steadily diminish over the next several seasons to the point where my sub 60 minute race time in college had ballooned to over 85 minutes.

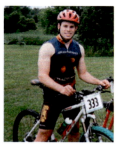

Adding 10-15 extra pounds to my frame made a big difference to my race times and not in a good way.

It wasn't just my race time that was suffering. My whole body felt sluggish and slow even on casual rides. Riding began to feel like a chore, and I started to favor other activities like rock climbing and hiking. I upgraded to a new mountain bike, but it didn't help much. Every year I grew more frustrated as riding felt more like a job rather than an enjoyable pastime. I even sold my road bike, and there were many weeks where that weekly training race was the only time I spent on the bike.

By the time I turned 30, I was about ready to throw in the towel, not just on riding but exercise in general. At that point, my body and mind felt beat up after 6 years of heavy lifting, and I felt like an old man as a collection of aches and pains greeting when I woke up each morning.

My frustrations lead me to consider bodyweight training as a way to take a break from the iron. As an experiment, I decided to give up the weights and focus on nothing but calisthenics for a full month. By the end of that 30 days, I looked and felt better than I had in years and decided to make bodyweight training the focus of my strength training routine.

The biggest surprise was discovering what calisthenics was doing for my lower body. I knew exercises like pull-ups and dips were great for my upper body, but I was concerned that my leg strength would suffer. How could I possibly ride, ski or hike well without squatting with a heavy barbell on my back?

I didn't need to worry though. After even a few months, my legs grew even stronger and more powerful than ever! By the end of that summer, I was back to riding without any pain or discomfort and my race times started to improve.

Over the next couple of years, I learned more about proper bodyweight training and things improved even more, both on and off the bike. I was completely free of any joint pain, and I was discovering some of that old explosive power I thought was long gone. Best of all, I was having a lot more fun on the bike again.

I continued to shave time off of those 20K races. Eventually, I even completed a couple of races in just under an hour. At this point, I was well over 30 pounds heavier than I was in college. I was also only riding 2-3 hours a week at most yet I was riding at the same pace I rode while in my prime. I had every reason to be as slow as ever, but I was the fastest I had been in years. The only difference was my practice of progressive bodyweight training.

Five years ago I moved from Vermont to Colorado to become a full-time personal trainer. Some of my clientele were riders and racers, so I started teaching them my tricks. It didn't take long for the positive feedback to start rolling in. People started telling me they had more strength, power, and endurance on the bike. Even better, they were more comfortable and less stiff after long rides. One of my clients accomplished a personal best on Strava on his first spring ride after training with me all winter. He rode faster on his first ride of the season than he had in all of the previous year!

I never expected calisthenics to help me, or my clients, ride so well. Knowing what I know now though it's fairly obvious why it works so well due to the following advantages.

#1 Efficiency

All training methods are only useful if you can consistently practice them. Maintaining a consistent training routine can be quite a challenge when a program demands a lot of time and energy from your already busy lifestyle.

Calisthenics has always been extremely efficient. You don't need to spend time and money to travel to and workout at a gym. In addition, each exercise provides multiple benefits relieving you from the burden of long and complicated workouts. All of this adds up to help you reap the most benefits from the least amount of work making it easier to train consistently for years on end.

#2 Holistic progression

The exercises in this book improve the three primary qualities you need to ride at your best. The first of these qualities is the muscular strength which lays down the foundation for your endurance, power and pedaling force.

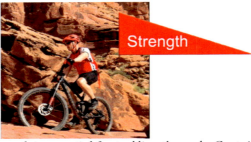

Raw muscular strength is essential for tackling the rocky Captain Ahab trail in Moab.

The second essential quality is mobility. Riding with stiff joints is like trying to ride with your brakes rubbing. Stiffness forces you work harder while robbing you of strength and power. Mobility is especially crucial for those who ride in the tucked or aero position on a road bike.

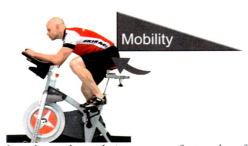

Hip mobility plays a key role in your comfort and performance.

Mobility also plays a vital role in your health and endurance. Stiff joints can tire you out while making you feel tight and sore after even short rides. You won't believe how much more comfortable you can ride when your joints are even a little more mobile.

The last quality of progression is stability. Riding with unstable joints is a lot like riding on an inefficient frame that soaks up your energy before it reaches the wheels. You can have the strongest and most mobile legs in the world, but you'll still lose a great deal of power to excessive motions that soak up your strength on each pedal stroke.

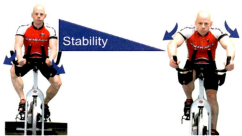

Unstable hips and shoulders create lateral motion or "winging" which leaks power and strength with each pedal stroke.

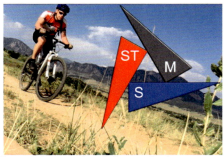

Combining strength, mobility, and stability is the key to a complete holistic conditioning program.

#3 Joint therapy

Your joints are the gatekeepers to your health and performance. It's a lot easier to achieve the results you want when your knees and lower back are not holding you back. Riding with joint pain is just as detrimental as riding with a flat tire.

The exercises in this book are hand-picked to not only strengthen your muscles, but your joints as well so you can stay healthy and resilient for years to come.

I could write a lot more about the endless benefits of calisthenics, but I would rather help you get started, so you can begin experiencing those benefits for yourself. Your journey begins on the next page.

Chapter 2

Three Moves For Ultimate Performance

It's easy to get lost in the seemingly infinite selection of exercises in the calisthenics universe. I once had a smartphone app that included over 300 push-up variations. All of this variety can make it difficult to filter out an effective training program from all the noise. That's why I've hand-picked just a few of the best exercises for their efficiency and useful functional carryover to cycling.

I like to think of the exercises in this book like the parts of a bicycle. While they all play an important role, some are more important than others. That's why I've listed these exercises in order of importance so you'll know what to focus on when time and energy are limited.

We start your journey with three incredibly effective and efficient exercises. Over 80% of the physical abilities you need to ride at your best comes from just these three exercises.

Movement #1 Squats (Frame)

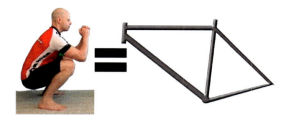

Like the frame on your bike, the squat is the foundational component of this program. The squatting motion is the most functional movement for cycling. The better you can squat the better you can ride. It's that simple.

There are a few reasons why squats are so ideal for cycling. The first is they require you to drive force directly downward just as you do while riding.

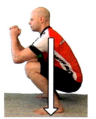 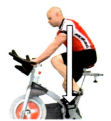

Squats apply force in a downward motion just like the downward motion of your pedal stroke.

The second benefit is they use a lot of strength and mobility in your hip joint. Weak and stiff hips are a prevalent issue in cycling, and they can severely handicap your performance.

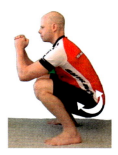 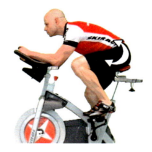

Lastly, squats require more stability than their seated weight machine counterparts. A lack of stability causes you to "leak" power just as you would while riding a bike with an inefficient frame or wheelset. The more stable your legs are, the more power you can bring to the pedals.

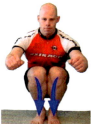 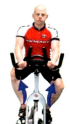

Stable hips help you use more of your strength, both in squats and on the bike.

The following squat exercises are designed to help you gradually build your strength, mobility, and stability in a progressive and balanced way.

Assisted Squats

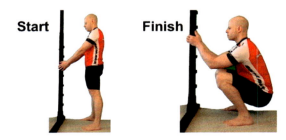

Assisted squats use your upper body to assist with the movement. Start by standing upright with your hands holding onto something sturdy and your arms bent. Drop down into a squat by pushing your knees forward so your hips can shift back and down toward your ankles. Make sure your weight stays in the middle of your foot. Be sure not to "drop" or fall into the squat as you lower yourself under control as low as possible.

After pausing at the bottom, drive your feet straight into the floor and stand back up while extending your hips, knees, and ankles.

Key points

This exercise gives you the opportunity to work on the mobility at your ankle, knee and hip joints while also maintaining tension in your calves, quads, and glutes through the full range of motion. Over time, you can work less on using your arms for support as your legs can take over.

Free Squats

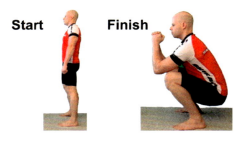

The next level of difficulty comes from doing full depth squats without any upper body assistance. At this stage, your legs are responsible for all of the strength, stability, and mobility for the exercise which will help you ride significantly better.

Key points

These are the bread-and-butter style squat, and I encourage you to use it as much as you can on a daily basis. Daily squat practice helps maintain joint mobility and prevents stiffness from developing in the hips, calves and lower back.

Notice how a deep unassisted squat requires you to pull yourself into the bottom position. This pulling motion uses the strength of the muscles in your shins, hamstrings and hip flexors.

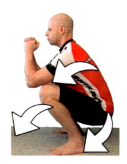

This pulling motion teaches your muscles how to pull through the bottom of each pedal stroke while using your hip flexors to pull your foot up and forward. This pulling motion smooths out your pedaling and prevents your quads from fatiguing too quickly.

Close Squats

Start 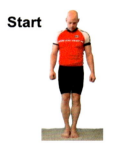 **Finish**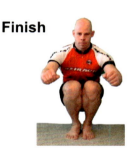

The width of your squat is a fun variable that can further challenge your strength, mobility, and stability. Moving your feet closer together can improve how well you squat, but it also creates more functional carry over to cycling. Common squat techniques involve squatting with the feet wider than shoulder width apart and with the feet and knees turned out. While this technique may be best for lifting heavy weights, cycling involves pointing your feet and knees forward.
Using a narrow squat stance isn't ideal for powerlifting, but it does help your muscles learn how to work on the bike optimally.

Just as with wider squats, feel free to experiment with close squats while using an upper body assist.

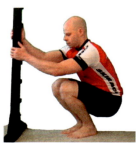

You can use some upper body assistance to get comfortable with deep close squats.

Key points

Most athletes tend to slightly round their back while squatting with their legs close together and this is perfectly fine. The old idea of keeping your back straight while squatting is a rule that mostly applies to squatting with an external weight. If you're not holding onto a weight, then feel free to allow your spine to flex forward a bit. As long as you are opening up the back of your hips, the stress on your lower back should be minimal.

Speaking of moving forward, try to push your knees forward so you can to keep your weight centered on your feet. This technique helps ease the stress on both your knees and your lower back by preventing your weight from falling too far back or reaching forward.

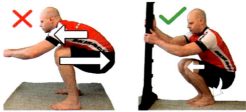

Allowing your knees to track forward will give your hips room to lower toward your heels. You'll have to bend your torso forward otherwise which can place more stress on your back.

Assist Single Leg Squats

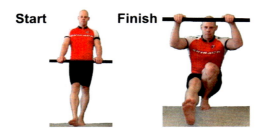

Single leg squats are the ultimate cycling exercise. They require the perfect mix of mobility, strength, and stability which carries over very well to cycling. The other benefit is they are a unilateral exercise meaning you work one leg at a time just like when riding. Unilateral leg exercises are also a great way to iron out any weaknesses and imbalances between your two legs that are holding you back.

As great as single leg squats are, they can be a tricky to learn. Even seasoned veterans of leg presses and back squats can find it hard to drop down on one leg and stand back up in a controlled manner.

The smart way to start single leg training is to use some upper body assistance while your legs get used to the exercise. You can do these many ways, but the basic idea is to hold onto something sturdy while you squat down on one leg. You can use your arms to help control your body as you squat down and pull yourself back up.

Doorways are often a good choice since they are sturdy and provide support along the full length of the squat. You can also adjust the amount of assistance you give yourself by where you stand in the doorway. The more you stand back, the more your arms can assist you. Standing slightly forward makes the exercise harder.

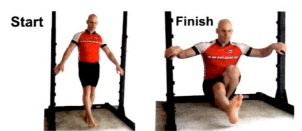

Doorways are an ideal way to practice single leg squats. You can easily adjust the difficulty by holding high or lower on the door frame or placing yourself behind or in the frame to adjust the difficulty.

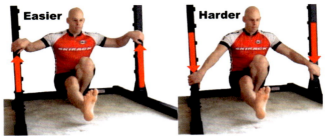

Placing your hands higher on the door frame makes the exercise easier. Grabbing lower on the frame makes it harder.

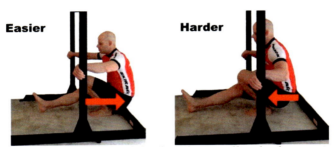

Placing your squatting foot behind the door frame will make the exercise easier while moving yourself more underneath the frame will make it harder.

Stairways are also an ideal place to practice single leg squats. The railings provide upper body assistance while the stairs slant down, so you don't need to pick up your non-squatting leg quite as high. The top step can also serve as a bit of support for your hips at the bottom of the squat and helps you know if your hips are tilting to one side at the bottom.

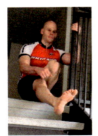 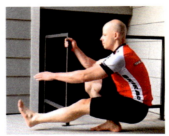

Railings, doorways and anything sturdy will work for a support with assisted single leg squats.

Be sure to hold onto something that's not going to move around on you like a piece of furniture that could tip over.

Your mission is to gradually reduce the amount of assistance you need during single leg squats so your squatting leg can provide the strength, mobility, and stability. There are many ways you can do this from using fewer fingers to hold on with each hand to only using one hand for support. You can also change the amount of assistance you use during the workout. You can do a few reps with one arm and then more reps with both to complete the set. However you progress, the basic idea is you'll be doing less work with your arms and more with your legs.

Key points

Single leg squats focus a little more on the hip stability, so it pays to work on keeping your muscles tense at the bottom of each rep. Avoid relaxing into the bottom of each squat while you let your upper body hold you in place.

Also, pay attention to any twisting and tilting you may do at the bottom of each rep. Try to keep your non-squatting leg pointing straight forward, and your legs close together. Doing this prevents stress on your joints while making your muscles work harder.

Free Single Leg Squats

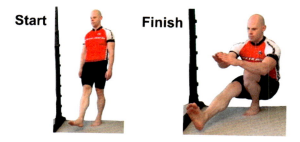

Unassisted single leg squats are the heavy hitters in the world of calisthenics leg training. Once you become proficient in single leg squats you'll have a lot more strength, stability and mobility in every pedal stroke. They leave nothing behind as single leg squats highlight even the smallest weaknesses in your lower body.

While they may look fancy or complicated, they are quite simple. You squat down and stand back up just as with any other squat motion. The only difference is you do it on one leg instead of two.

Key points

Learning to do single leg squats is a lot like learning to ride a bike. It's an enriching activity but learning how to do it proficiently is just the start. There is always room to improve no matter how proficient you become in this exercise.

The most significant areas you can strive to improve are stability and mobility. Make it your mission to move with as much confidence and control as you would have on two legs. I'm talking no excessive movement or shaking whatsoever from one rep to the next. Try to make it look easy.

Progressing Beyond Free Single Leg Squats

You can develop even more strength by dropping your hips lower over time. Every millimeter of depth you gain requires much more strength and control. The ultimate test would be to stand up on one leg from a seated position. Now that's some serious lower body strength!

Clasping your hands together and pulling them closer to your torso is another way to make single leg squats more difficult. This modification causes your weight to shift back a bit and makes your squatting leg work much harder.

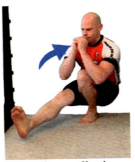

Pulling your hands closer to your chest will take your squat skills to a whole new level!

Movement #2 Bridges (Wheels)

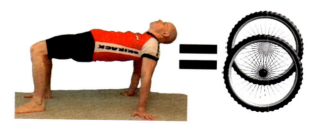

Just like the wheels on your bike, bridges play two significant roles in helping you ride faster and safer. First, they strengthen the muscles in the back of your legs like your hamstrings and glutes. These muscles are often neglected in cycling as the quads and calves tend to get the lion's share of attention. Strengthening the muscles in the back of your legs can smooth out your pedal stroke while adding power. They also keep muscle imbalances at bay and can help prevent excess stress on the knees.

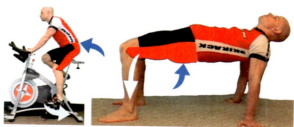

The hamstrings and glutes play an important role in pulling your leg down and back (white arrow) which helps drive your hips forward (blue arrow).

The second benefit of bridging is it helps reverse the detrimental effects of sitting for long periods of time. Sitting makes the muscles on the front of your body tight and weak while turning off the muscles on the backside. These muscle habits not only hold you back on the bike but also cripple your posture and increase your risk for chronic injury. Bridging is the exact antidote to the issues associated with sitting. It wakes up and strengthens the muscles on your backside while stretching and opening the up the muscles up front.

Lying Bridges

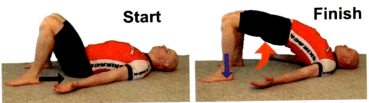

Start by pulling your heels toward your hips to turn on your hamstrings. Then press your feet straight into the floor while lifting your hips.

Lying bridges are a gentle exercise that helps your hamstrings and glutes wake up while stretching out the front of your hips. They are also a great way to loosen up after a long ride, so you don't feel as stiff the following day. This exercise is usually done for reps by lifting and lowering your hips off the floor repeatedly, but lifting and holding and isometric for time is also very common.

Key points

All bridges in this book are hip-dominant movements. Focus on lifting yourself up with the tension in your hamstrings and glutes. Excess tension in the lower back is a sign that you're not pulling into the top of the bridge with the muscles on the back of your legs. It helps to squeeze your shoulder blades together and press them down toward your hips. This additional back tension keeps your spine stable, so you lift with your hips instead of your lower back.

You might feel your hamstrings cramp up the first time you perform this exercise. Cramping often happens when the hamstrings are new to the workload of the exercise, and they need some time to get used to the move. In this case, don't lift your hips up quite as high.

Cramping hamstrings are also a sign that your glutes are not holding enough tension to do their part. If this is the case, try holding your hips just off the floor and practice tensing up your glutes without moving. This isometric technique helps you learn how to engage your glutes and make them work more during the exercise as well as on the bike.

Table Bridges

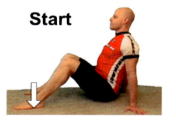 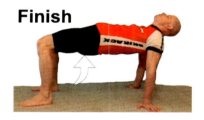

Table bridges are an excellent exercise for training your hips through a large range of motion while stretching the muscles in the chest and shoulders which are typically tight for cyclists. Start off sitting on the floor with your hands behind your hips. Lift up your chest while keeping tension in your back. Drive your hips up to form a table position. Pause at the top and then lower your hips back to the floor. Be sure to maintain tension in your hamstrings, glutes and back as you lower yourself down.

Key points

Table bridges can feel like they are more about mobility than strength especially if your upper body is tight. You may struggle a bit to lift your hips very high and create a dip in the middle of your "table" position. Struggling to move in a full range of motion is perfectly normal and shouldn't discourage you. Just continue to pull your shoulders back while trying to drive up you're your hips while using whatever range you can manage. You'll find your upper body will loosen up in time.

Straight Bridges

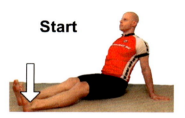 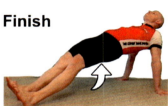

Straight bridges, or reverse planks, are a useful strength exercise for your glutes and hamstrings while improving stability in your shoulders. They don't require quite as much upper body mobility as table bridges because you won't be lifting your hips as high. Nevertheless, this is still a valuable shoulder exercise and a great way to reverse the effects of sitting for long periods of time. They work pretty much the same way with pressing your heels into the floor and using your glutes and hamstrings to lift up your hips.

Key points

This exercise requires a lot of tension control in the hamstrings and glutes to lift up and support your hips. You may find your lower back wants to do most of the work if your glutes or hamstrings are not strong enough. If that's the case, bend your knees to make the exercise easier so you can improve the tension control in the back of your legs. As always, keep your shoulder blades down and back to keep your spine stable.

Cross Bridges

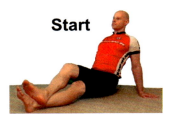
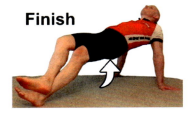

The three bridges I've mentioned are in progressive order with lying bridges being the easiest; table bridges are intermediate and straight bridges are the most difficult.

You can also progress each of these hip bridges by shifting more weight onto one side, so one leg needs to work harder than the other. The first way you can do this is with cross bridges where you cross your ankles. This position places more weight on the foot that's on the floor while the top leg acts as an assist.

Key points

Be sure to do the same number of reps on each leg to keep your development even. Place your working leg close to your centerline so you won't have to twist or torque your upper body around too much.

Single Leg Bridges

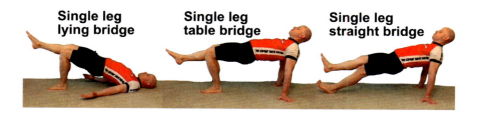

The next step in difficulty is the single leg bridge which you can do with all three bridge variations. This exercise places most of your weight on one leg making your hamstring and glutes work incredibly hard. It also requires a lot of hip and core stability which significantly improves your pedaling efficiency.

Key points

The most common question I get regarding single leg bridges is what do you do with the non-working leg? Some athletes like to kick up the non-working leg like a can-can dancer to use momentum and make the exercise easier. I find it's much better to stick the leg straight out in front of you and allow it to raise and lower with your hips. This technique will not only add extra weight to the exercise but also prevents momentum from making the exercise easier. If you find the single leg variation is too difficult, try going back to the cross bridges and place a little less weight on the crossing leg to dial in the appropriate level of resistance.

Movement #3 Planks (Drive Train)

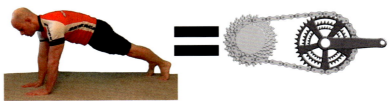

Your core and anterior chain help you transfer power just like your drivetrain transfers your leg power into your wheels.

You can have the best frame and wheel-set in the world, but you still won't go anywhere if you can't get any power through the whole system. Just like the drivetrain on your bike feeds power to the wheels your core helps transfer power through your body and bike.

Planks are a great exercise for training all of the muscles on the front of your body to work as a complete unit. While typically thought of as an abdominal or core exercise, planks also improve hip and shoulder stability. They are also an efficient way to train your muscles to work in a similar way you use them on the bike. Planks essentially use the muscles on the front of your body to pull the floor together to create stability. The same muscles work in a very similar way when riding as your hips, and abs work to create stability between your hands and your hips. Such stability is crucial when climbing as you work to "pull" your bike under you with each pedal stroke.

Knee Plank

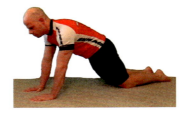

The knee plank is an excellent place to start to learn the technical details of the plank. It's not the most challenging exercise, but it's not meant to be. Instead, this is a helpful way to improve the strength and mobility in your wrists while learning how to pull yourself into the plank while tilting your hips back.

Key points

The knee plank is an opportunity to learn how to use your abs to hold your hips tucked in a hollow body position. Slightly tilting your hips back to gently round you back will engage your abs in a very similar way to when you're on the bike.

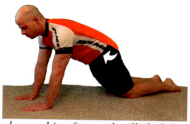

Using your abs to slightly tuck your hips forward will slightly arch your back just like when on the bike.

It's also a good way to learn how to pull your upper body and lower body toward each other as if you're trying to squeeze the floor together. Doing this will ensure you're using the muscles on the front of your body to provide the support you need on the bike.

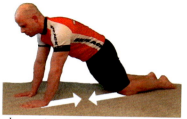

Pulling the floor together helps maintain supportive tension along the front of your body.

Toe Plank

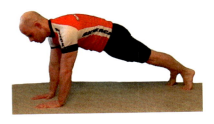

This exercise is the classic plank position many people are familiar with. You can do this on your arms or your hands with each position offering a unique benefit. The elbow position positions your torso more horizontal to gravity which slightly increases the resistance of the exercise. Doing a plank on your hands makes it easier to adjust the position of your arms while improving the strength and mobility of your wrists.

Key points

While often considered a "core" exercise, the toe plank is a full body move so it pays to tense up as many muscles as you can. Keep your shoulders and lats tense to stabilize your upper body. The tension then flows into your abs and hips before moving into the tension of your glutes. Lastly, keep your quads and shin muscles tense to complete a solid plank that's strong and stable.

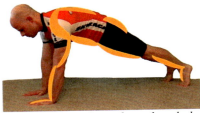

The classic plank position uses tension throughout the whole body including the back, shoulders, glutes and quads.

Stretch Plank

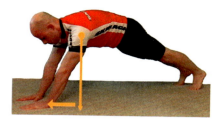

Stretch planks are the next step in the plank progressions and involve extending your body to make the plank more difficult. Reaching your hands forward so they are not under your shoulders is the easiest way to accomplish this.

I recommend starting with a kneeling plank to set your muscle tension and then lift your knees off the floor to move into a toe plank. Once you're in the toe plank, slide your feet back until you've reached the length you want and hold.

Key points

The tricky part of stretching planks is to still pull the floor together between your hands and feet instead of trying to brace yourself by pushing the floor apart. You may also find pushing straight into the floor to be a viable option as well.

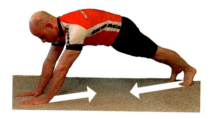

Also, pay attention to your breathing and avoid holding your breath which can be common while holding an isometric exercise.

Cross Plank

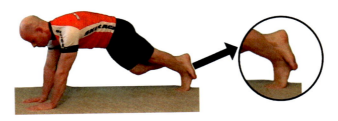

Cross planks are similar to the cross leg bridges in the last chapter. The most significant difference is you can cross either your arms or legs to bring some variety to the exercise. Both variations are challenging and slightly alter where the resistance is in your body. Crossing your hands makes your upper body work slightly harder while crossing at the ankles makes your abs and hips work harder. Crossing your legs during a knee plank isn't possible, but you can bring your knees together to create a similar effect. Experiment with which style appeals to you.

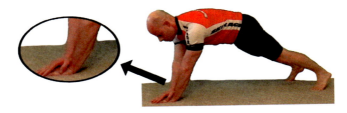

Key points

Just like with cross leg bridges, keep your hands or feet are close to your centerline to avoid excessive torque on your spine and hips. Be sure to practice for an equal amount of time on each side to avoid developing imbalances.

Single Arm/ Leg Plank

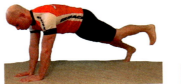 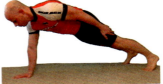

Single arm and leg planks are a challenging technique that can do wonders for your shoulder and hip stability while seriously ramping up the resistance on your core. While these planks are challenging, they are quite simple. Just pick one foot or hand off the floor and keep it close to your centerline. You don't need to lift them very high. Just an inch or two will do the trick.

Key points

Just like with cross planks, be sure to keep the single supporting hand or foot close to your centerline. Pay attention to any twisting your hips and shoulders might do with an uneven load. Such twisting should be safe unless you have any injuries or lower back issues, but you'll get more from the exercise with minimal movement to the side.

Mountain Climbers

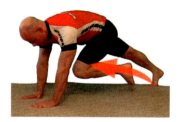

Mountain climbers are essentially alternating single leg planks that improve your ability to drive your knees toward your chest. These are very good for developing not only core strength but also hip strength and mobility.

Key points

Many athletes practice mountain climbers at a fast pace sort of like when pedaling in a sprint. A quick cadence is great for building explosive power, but I recommend using a slow tempo to improve your strength and hip mobility. Try to take 1-2 seconds to lift your knee toward your chest and hold it there for 3-5 seconds before placing your foot back into the plank position. Repeat with the other leg.

Chapter 3

Two Moves For Total Control

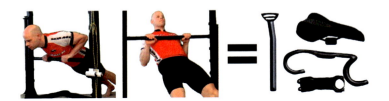

These moves condition the major muscle groups in your upper body. While they may not play a significant role in turning your pedals, they do a lot to influence your body position and bike handling abilities just like the components on your bicycle.

Both of these exercises have many variations ranging from very easy to insanely difficult. Since this is a book for cyclists, and not bodybuilders or calisthenics sport athletes, I've only included the basic progressive versions of both exercises. Once you can perform 2-3 sets of 20 on the most challenging variation of each, you'll have all the strength you need to ride at your best.

Check out my book, Smart Bodyweight Training if you would like to challenge yourself beyond these progressions.

Push-Ups

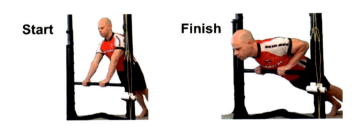

Almost all cycling positions involve some version of an isometric push-up. The muscles in the chest, shoulders, and triceps play a crucial role in helping you control your bike over technical terrain. They also work hard when you crouch down low in a more aerodynamic position on a road bike.

Progressing your push-up is as simple as adjusting your angle to gravity. The more upright you are, the easier the exercise will be. Moving your hands close to the floor shifts more of your weight onto your hands so your pushing muscles will work harder.

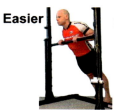 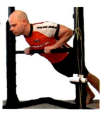 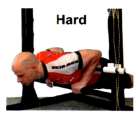

Key points

Flaring elbows is a common issue amongst cyclists. Flaring happens when the muscles in the upper body fail to bring the elbows in and allows the chest to fall forward. This riding position can create more work for your back and stress the spine. It also severely compromises your aerodynamic profile on a road bike.

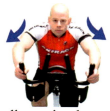

To combat this, try to squeeze your elbows in close to your body while performing push-ups. Keep your hands about a foot apart and tuck your elbows in to your sides. Also be sure to keep your shoulder blades down and close together. These technical adjustments will help bring more tension to your muscles while removing stress from your joints.

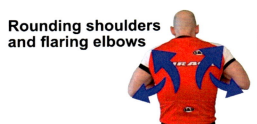 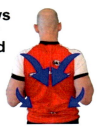

Rounding shoulders and flaring elbows   **Pulling elbows and shoulder blades inward**

Keep in mind that push-ups are a moving plank so try to keep tension in your back, abs, hips, glutes, and quads just as you would with a standard plank.

Lastly, experiment with your hand position both with how wide your hands are and how far forward you place them relative to your torso. I recommend keeping your hands at the same width you would use while riding your bike. You can use a tape measure and make marks on the floor to ensure you're using a consistent width for each set.

While you reach your hands out in front of you on a bike, you'll probably be better off keeping your hands under your chest when doing push-ups. Some athletes find they are most comfortable keeping their wrists at the bottom of their chest. Experiment with subtle shifts in where you place your hands to see what's best for you.

Rows

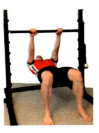 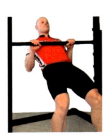

Start   **Finish**

It may not always feel like it, but your back muscles work very hard when riding your bike. This is especially the case when you accelerate and climb up a steep hill. Strong back muscles also prevent you from hunching over the handlebars which saps your energy and creates stress in the middle of your spine.

Bodyweight rows are an excellent back exercise because they offer a lot of carryover to cycling without placing a lot of stress along your spine. You can progress this exercise the same way you progress push-ups. Use a more upright posture to decrease the resistance on your back and arms. The lower your angle to gravity the more resistance you'll place on your muscles.

More upright is easier
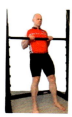

Lower and more reclined is harder
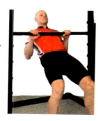

Rowing is one of the few bodyweight exercises you'll need some equipment to use. You may be able to find some monkey bars or ledges at the local playground or gymnasium. My preference has always been to use a suspension trainer or set of gymnastics rings. These are much easier to use for adjusting your angle to gravity. You can also set them up at home and take them with you when traveling.

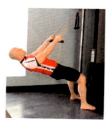 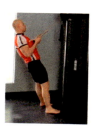 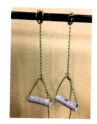

You can find a variety of suspension trainers on the internet, or you can make your own from a rope or nylon straps. I have a complete description of how to make two different trainers in my book Smart Bodyweight Training.

Key points

Like with push-ups, flaring elbows are also common with pulling exercises. You'll find you get more value in each rep if you work hard to squeeze your arms in tight to your sides as you pull yourself up.

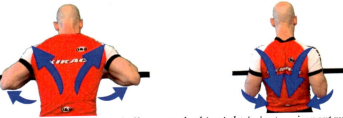

Keeping your shoulder blades and elbows tucked in tight is just as important during rows as it is during push-ups.

Chapter 4

Accessory Moves

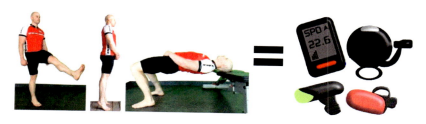

The following exercise are accessory moves to shore up weak points and help prevent a few aches and pains from holding you back. These are not a make-or-break exercise any more than a cycling computer, or seat pack would make or break your ability to ride, but they are great to have when you want or need them. Feel free to adopt and discard them as you wish.

Calf Raises

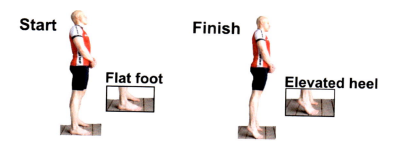

We cyclists are known for our calves because we work these muscles so much while riding. Calf muscles work especially hard when using clipless pedals. Some say they don't train their calves because they work so much on the bike. I say I work my calves *because* they are used so much on the bike. Plus, it's not like they take a lot of time and energy to train in a workout.

I recommend balanced standing calf raises. Just stand with your weight equally distributed between both feet and tense up all of the muscles in your core and lower body. Press into the balls of your feet and lift your heels off the floor. Pause at the top and bring your heels back on the floor under control. Let your heels "kiss" the ground lightly before lifting yourself back up fro another rep.

Doing calf raises without upper body support builds strength as well as stability for greater pedaling efficiency. While you may not need much ankle stability on the bike, it can come in handy when you need to hike-a-bike over a tricky section of trail or when running and jumping in cyclocross.

Some experts advocate that you always do calf raises on a ledge so your heels can drop down below the level of your toes. This technique is an excellent option for increasing the mobility of your ankle, but it often requires holding onto something for balance.

My experience has been that most riders benefit more from improving their calf stability first and mobility second. I've also seen many folks do calf raises on a ledge, but their heel doesn't drop down much further than if they were standing on the floor. Experiment with what version works best for you.

Leg Raises

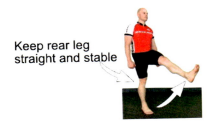
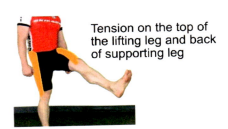

Keep rear leg straight and stable

Tension on the top of the lifting leg and back of supporting leg

You're only as strong as your legs, and your legs are only as strong as your hips. Unfortunately, stiff and weak hips are a big problem for cyclists due to the sitting position we use on the bike. Progressive squats and bridges can do wonders for your hips. Throw in some mountain climbers or single leg planks and you're 99% there. Still, you may find your hips need a little extra attention from time to time. These two exercises improve your hip strength, stability, and mobility well beyond what you'll need on the bike.

The first hip exercise is to stand with both feet close together and your legs straight. Lift one leg straight out in front of you while keeping your other leg locked and your torso upright.

This exercise works both the front and back of your hips in opposition to one another. The front hip is working on the lifting leg while the back and inside hip are working on the supporting leg. This exercise also helps stretch the hamstring of both legs.

The second hip exercise is to lift one leg to the side while tilting your body in the opposite direction. Start with your feet close together and angled about 30 degrees away from the direction you'll lift your leg. Lift the outside leg straight out while tilting away with your torso. This technique works the outer hips of both your lifting and supporting leg.

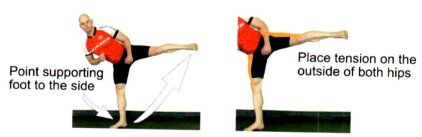

Point supporting foot to the side

Place tension on the outside of both hips

Neck Bridges

Weak neck muscles can quickly become fatigued which can stress your upper back and cause headaches.

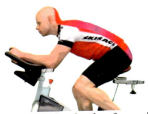

Riding naturally places stress on the backside of your body with your lower back and neck receiving most of the stress.

Simple neck bridges can do wonders for your back and neck strength so it's easier to ride while looking up. Lean your upper back against a sturdy wall with a cloth or towel against the back of your head. Tighten the muscles on the back of your body, like a bridge, and tense the muscles in your upper back and neck to hold yourself up. You can also switch around and do this for the muscles on the front of your neck.

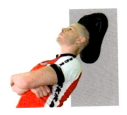 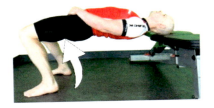

A more advanced variation of this is to do neck bridges against a weight bench or piece of furniture. Just sit on the floor with the back of your head against a study padded surface. Lift your hips up by driving into your heels just like with normal hip bridges.

Both of these exercises are isometric exercises where you'll hold for 20-30 seconds for each set.
Also, be careful the first time you do this exercise as your neck muscles may not be used to the stress of applying resistance to them.

Chapter 5

Simple Stretches For An Easier Ride

One of the benefits of calisthenics training is that it builds a decent level of mobility in you joints as you strengthen your muscles. Deep squats and bridges are a couple of the best examples. While some muscles are working others are stretching all the while maintaining stability around the joints. This sort of thing is what the old-time strength athletes used to call subtle strength. This subtle strength isn't just about stretching a muscle, but teaching your muscles how to be strong, stable and flexible all at the same time. This trifecta of qualities will not only make the body stronger but more resilient as well.

It's for this reason that I gave up static stretching years ago. I've been a martial artist since the age of 10 and have done a lot of stretching over the past 30 years. Looking back, I can honestly say that passive stretching never improved my flexibility or performance very much. It didn't even prevent me from getting hurt either. I used to pull muscles in my back and lower body on an almost weekly basis. Thankfully, everything changed when I discovered the value of subtle strength. Since then, I've improved the flexibility around every joint in my body and injuries are almost nonexistent despite abstaining from stretching for over 10 years.

I've come to believe the ultimate test of a body's functional abilities isn't how mobile and flexible it is when it's all stretched out and warmed up. Anyone can feel loose and move better after an extensive warm up. The real test is how loose and mobile your joints are from a stone-cold start. I'm talking wake yourself up at 3 am on a cold January morning and see how you feel at that moment. If your flexibility and mobility routine is working, you should feel looser and move easier even when waking up in the morning. If that's not the case, then maybe it's time to give subtle strength a serious try.

Most of the exercises you've already learned develop a good deal of subtle strength, but here are some of my other favorites that can help you even more.

Behind Back Stretch

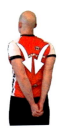 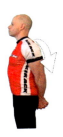 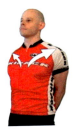

This stretch is a simple way to work the muscles in your back while stretching the muscles in the front of your torso. It's especially useful for relieving shoulder stress that can accumulate on road rides. All you need to do is clasp your hands behind you while pushing your shoulders down and back.

You can also slightly arch your back to stretch out your abs. Just be sure not to strain your back by trying to force yourself through the stretch.

Snow Angels

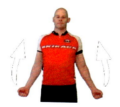 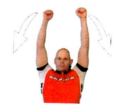

This simple exercise mimics the classic motion you made with your arms while making snow angels as a kid. Just stretch your arms back as far as you can with your palms facing forward and move them up and up and down in a smooth motion. Do your best to keep pulling your arms back without arching your back or letting your hands move forward. Note that you can do this stretch both laying down, which is a little easier, and standing which is a little more difficult.

Deep Wide Squat

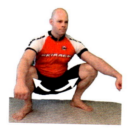

The squat variations in this book are beneficial for opening up your hips but what if you want to go a little further? We cyclists are typically both tight and weak on the inner thigh so this squat variation can help both strengthen and stretch those muscles.

Getting into a deep squat is as simple as pointing your feet and knees outward and then squatting down. The wider your stance is and the deeper you squat, the greater the stretch.

Be sure not to relax into the bottom of the squat. You want to place at least some tension in your muscles to build that subtle strength rather than a passive stretch.

Cross Leg Sit

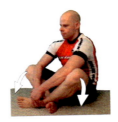

Sitting with your legs crossed is a useful hip mobility drill to do after a ride. Sit down, cross your ankles, and pull your torso forward while gently pushing your hips down with your elbows. Try pulling your knees close to the floor with the strength of your hips.

You may want to sit with your back against a wall if your hips are not quite strong or mobile enough to hold yourself up. You can push off the wall with your hands, but you'll get more benefit from pulling yourself forward with your hip muscles.

Twist and Hold

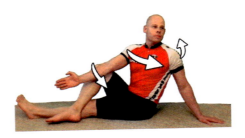

Rotational mobility can do wonders to relieve stress that builds up in the hips and back while on the bike. You can twist in both a sitting and lying position.

For sitting stretches sit with both legs out in front and bend one knee so that one foot is flat on the floor. Reach out with the opposite arm and push that arm against the outside of the knee while placing the other arm behind you for support.

From there, sit up straight while using the muscles in the torso to gently twist toward the hand that's on the floor. Hold for several moments, release and repeat on the other side.

The lying down version uses gravity to assist your muscles in the twisting motion. To do this, lay on one side on the floor with your top leg extended out in front. Place both arms straight out in front of your torso with your palms together.

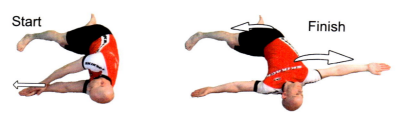

Slide your top hand forward a few inches and gently reach around until your hand is pointing behind you. Try not to let your extended foot lift off the floor. Hold this position for several moments and lower your hand toward your hip to release the stretch. Switch to the other side and repeat.

As with all stretches be sure to keep breathing in calm, deep breaths. Use your muscles to pull yourself into the stretch but don't try to force the range of motion beyond a moderate stretch. Your muscles will open up at their own pace and trying to force them can make them tighter.

How often should you stretch?

I recommend doing some form of subtle strength drills on a daily basis. Simply hold a stretch for 20-30 seconds once or twice a day whenever you find it to be convenient. You don't need to set aside much time to dedicate to stretching. Doing even a little every day brings you more benefit than doing a long stretching routine a few times a week.

Chapter 6

Routines and Training Tips For Success

A good routine should be simple, efficient and require only a minimal amount of time and energy. Think of your workout sort of like taking a post-ride shower. It's a regular habit that helps you look and feel your best, but it's a means to an end, and that's it. It's not the sort of thing you should have to plan your whole day or week around. That's why I created some simple routines that range in cost and benefit. Just pick the one that's suitable for your needs and resources.

Fully Rigid Routine

The fully rigid routine is like a bare-bones single speed mountain bike. It's just the core essentials of the primary three exercises you need to ride better.

> **Fully Rigid**
> 2 Rounds of:
> Squats
> Bridges
> Planks

Perform one exercise after the next with minimal rest between each exercise and rest 60-90 seconds between your first and second round.

Do this routine 2x a week on non-consecutive days (i.e., Monday and Thursday). Complete the whole workout in a circuit where you do one set of squats, bridges, and planks before returning to the squats for the second round. Bear in mind that the 2 rounds of each circuit refer to working rounds and don't include any warm up sets.

Hard Tail Routine

Built for speed but with a little extra up front, the Hard Tail routine is a full body routine that focuses on the primary three while ensuring your upper body gets the attention it deserves.

> **Hard Tail**
> **2-3 sets of:**
> 1a Squats   2a Plank
> 1b Push-ups   2b Bridge
>   2c Row

Perform this routine 2x a week on non-consecutive days (i.e., Monday and Thursday). Complete the squats and push-ups together in a superset with 60 seconds of rest between each round. Then move onto the second superset of bridges, rows, and planks as a circuit with 60 seconds of rest between each round. Be sure to perform the same number of rounds for both sets of exercises.

Full Suspension Routine

Like a fully tricked out ride, the Full Suspension routine is for those who want to make sure they are optimizing their strength and conditioning training. It includes a full load of exercises to ensure you're as ready as ever for your next century or the biggest race of the season.

> **Full Suspension**
>
> **2-3 Rounds of:**
>
> 1a Squats   2a Push-Up
> 1b Bridges   2b Plank
> 1c Calf Raise 2c Row
>
> 3a Neck work
> 3b Hip work

Perform the full workout 2x a week on non-consecutive days. Complete each circuit before moving onto the next with 60-90 seconds of rest in between each round.

Workout Tips

Like riding, training is often more art than science, and there's a lot of room for flexibility if you want to make any changes to suit your needs. With that said, there are a few tips I've picked up over the years that can help you get the most out of your workouts.

#1 Don't train to a high level of muscle fatigue

Training for strength and performance is different than training to build muscle. This program was designed to improve your ability to ride a bike over getting jacked. Besides, adding a bunch of extra muscle can weigh you down on the bike.

There are several differences between training for performance vs. muscle, but the biggest one is how you manage fatigue. Training to build muscle is often characterized by pushing your muscles to contract until they are very fatigued and tired. Some experts advocate doing the exercise until you can no longer perform one more rep. This approach is great for building muscle, but it's not the way to train if you want to stay light and strong on the bike.

That's why I recommend stopping a set with a few reps in the tank. You still want to push yourself, make sure you're saving a little "juice" in the muscle. Doing this still teaches your muscles to be stronger without leaving you too drained for an upcoming ride while preventing unwanted weight gain.

#2 Challenge the qualities you want to improve

There is no one best or perfect way to exercise even for a seemingly specific activity like cycling. All of the exercises in this book are simply tools, and your results depend on how you use them.

The most basic way to think about how to use your exercises is you gain the physical ability you challenge. If an exercise challenges your strength, you get stronger. If it challenges your stability, you'll improve balance. If it challenges endurance, you'll improve stamina and so on.

Don't get too hung up on what the supposed best rep range is or how many sets the experts claim are best. The most important thing is to adjust the difficulty of your exercise to challenge the performance qualities you want to improve. As a general rule, most athletes thrive from doing 6-10 reps of each exercise for 2-3 sets. Feel free to adjust your training any way you like to focus on the aspects of performance that are important to you. If stamina is your goal then you may want to see how many squats you can do in 5 minutes or how long you can hold a plank for. If you want to get stronger, adjust your technique so you're only able to perform 3-6 reps or hold a position for 15 seconds. If stability is your deal then you may want to try doing leg raises on one leg without any upper body support or try using one leg while doing push-ups.

#3 Keep a workout log

Successful training requires three simple things and keeping a workout log goes a long way toward ensuring you have all three in every training session.

The first thing you need is a stable workout routine. Having your workout plan written down ensures your workouts don't become a mess of random exercises and movements. Writing down what you plan to do, like 3 sets of squats and bridges every Sunday, makes it all the more likely that you'll stick to that plan on a consistent weekly basis.

The second important variable in successful training is progression. You don't get faster or stronger by doing a "correct" workout routine. You get faster and stronger by doing your current routine progressively better over time.

Progress often happens in small, and very forgettable steps from one workout to the next. If you do 10 table bridges how do you know if that's an improvement over what you did before? Did you do 9 last time or was it 12? If you're not sure what you did in your last workout you can't be sure you've made progress. If you're not sure if you've made progress, you won't know if your workout was effective or not. You may even be going backward and not even know it!

The last essential variable is analysis. Frequently, progress isn't as simple as just doing one more rep or shaving a few seconds off a race time. It's often hiding amongst the details of your performance, and it may take a moment of reflection to find it. Maybe you can increase your range of motion on the last few reps in a set. Perhaps you can improve by breathing through the rep rather than holding your breath. Taking a moment to write down what you did can help your mind reflect on what you can do to improve next time. Whatever you find, writing it down ensures you won't forget what to work on in your next workout.

The primary lesson is this; don't entrust your future progress to your memory. Human recollection is a fickle and unreliable thing. You wouldn't want to ride a bike you can't rely on, so why entrust the success of your conditioning to your memory? Taking just a few minutes to get things down on paper can make all the difference in the world.

#4 Plan your workouts around your rides and races

It doesn't make much sense to spend your best efforts in a squat workout only to feel like your legs are as heavy as lead when you get on the bike. For that reason, it pays to plan your workouts, so they don't impede your ride time.

If at all possible, try to leave 48 hours between your workouts and rides. This strategy can help your muscles recover so your rides don't compromise your workouts and vice versa.

If your ride schedule doesn't allow at least a full day between rides and workouts, plan to make your workouts lighter and less stressful before your rides. Just do one or two moderate sets and stop each set when you're about 75% fatigued. Not only will this help keep your legs fresh for your ride, but it can also fire them up and make them even more ready to ride.

Workouts that happen soon after a ride or race should also be on the light side, so you don't create excessive fatigue in your already tired muscles. A light workout can help in recovery by enhancing blood flow to the tired muscles which reduces soreness and stiffness in the day or two after your ride.

The most significant difference with workouts before a ride vs. workouts after is it's better to take it easy the day before a ride or race. Workouts that happen after a ride should be on the light side, but you can push harder if you feel like it. As you know, the amount of fatigue from a ride can vary greatly so play it by ear and listen to your body.

It's Time To Ride!

Well, my friend, the trails are calling, so it's time to wrap this sucker up and head out for a ride. At this point, you now understand more about how to use your bodyweight to ride stronger and faster than ever. While I've included a good amount of info on these pages, there's always more to learn and discover about calisthenics. To learn more you can also find videos on any of the exercises in this book on the Red Delta Project YouTube channel and at www.RedDeltaProject.com.

As a reminder, you can also learn more about progressive calisthenics training in my book **Smart Bodyweight Training** where you'll also find some information on performance nutrition, core training and DIY calisthenics equipment. Speaking of calisthenics equipment; many of the photos in this book featured an apparatus called the **Bodyweight Master**. I'm a huge fan of this calisthenics home gym and I highly recommend it. You can Learn more about these resources at reddeltaproject.com.

May the wind always be at your back,

- Matt Schifferle

Made in the USA
Lexington, KY
06 February 2019